October 2019

HOPE

Brain Injury
HOPE
MAGAZINE
"Supporting the
Brain Injury Community"

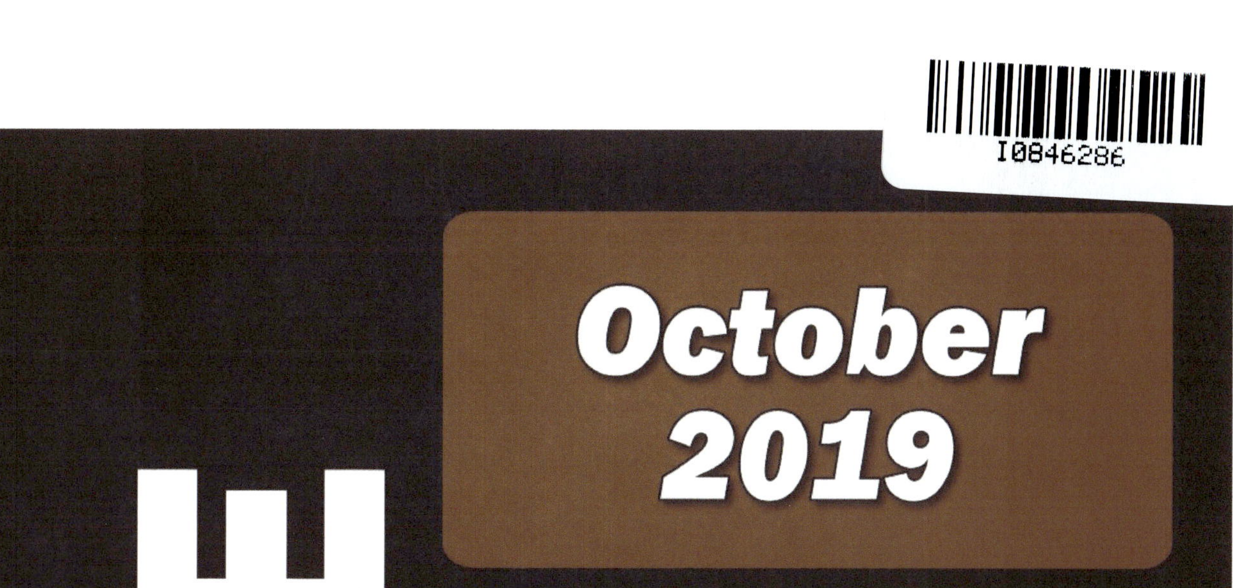

Welcome

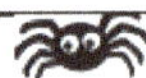

HOPE MAGAZINE

Serving the Brain Injury Community Since 2015

October 2019

Publisher
David A. Grant

Editor
Sarah Grant

Our Contributors

Patrick Brigham
Lynn Kaye
Vanessa R. Garza
David A. Grant
Martin Johnson
D. A. "Bo" Nanna
Rebecca Veenstra
Courtney Williams

Welcome to the October 2019 Issue of HOPE Magazine

Fall is in full swing here in New England. Leaves begin their yearly migration from green to red, yellow and orange. It's a transition season here as we say goodbye to summer and brace for another winter.

In a very true sense, brain injury follows a similar path as we transition from our pre-injury lives into who we become after brain injury. For most of us, the change began in an instant, but learning to live life anew is very much a lifelong and transitional process.

Next month marks nine years since my own brain injury. They have been nine of the most bittersweet years of my existence. There have been stunning gains – gains that dramatically exceeded my predicted outcome. And like most anyone, I have experienced gut wrenching losses. It's all part of our shared human experience.

This month we again have the privilege of bringing you stories from caregivers as well as TBI and ABI survivors. It remains our hope that you see some of your own life in the stories we share, and that in that seeing, you feel less alone, and that you come away from it knowing that you can indeed live a meaningful life after brain injury.

I wish you peace.

David A. Grant
Publisher

Contents

What's Inside This Issue

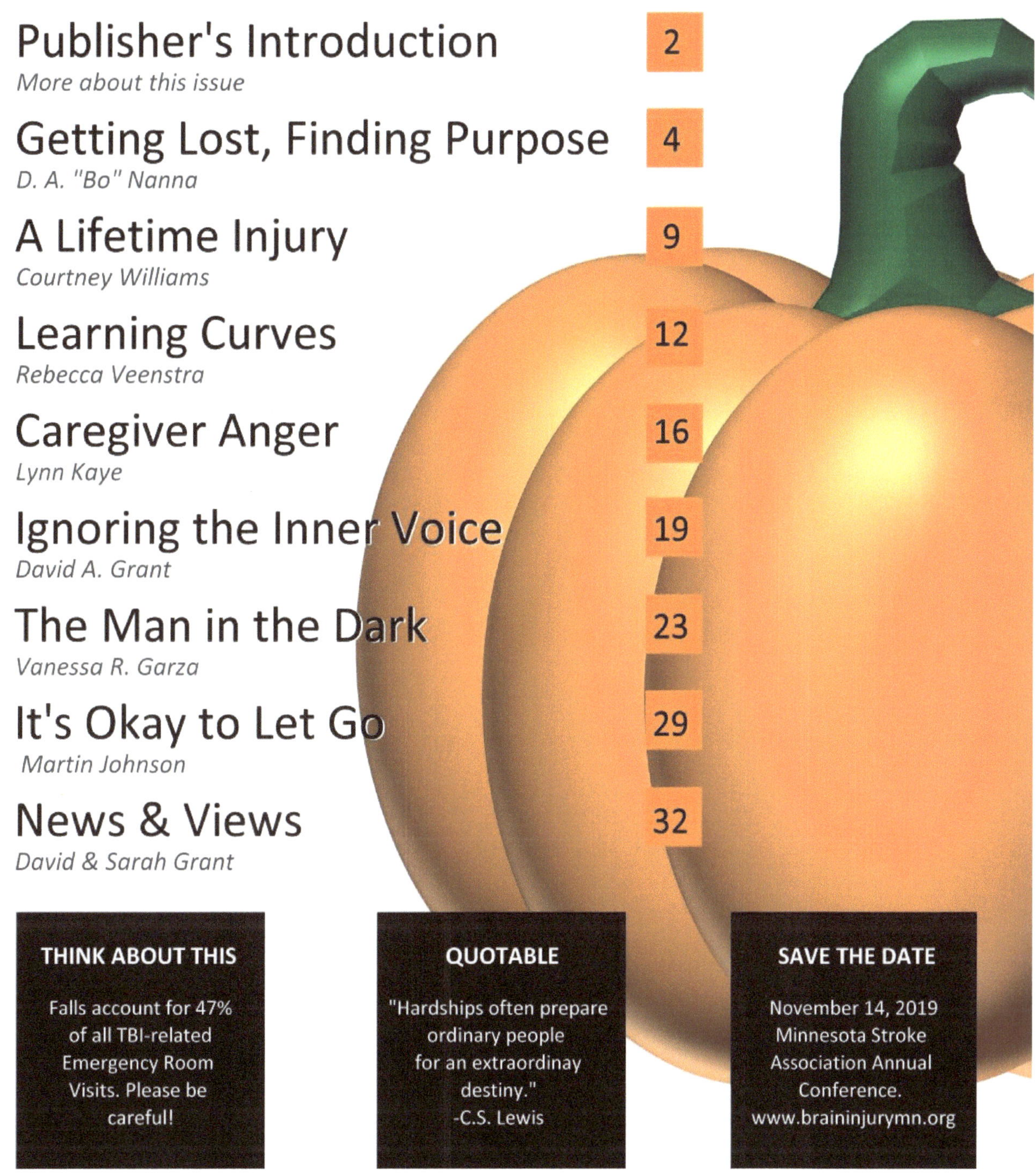

THINK ABOUT THIS

Falls account for 47% of all TBI-related Emergency Room Visits. Please be careful!

QUOTABLE

"Hardships often prepare ordinary people for an extraordinay destiny."
-C.S. Lewis

SAVE THE DATE

November 14, 2019 Minnesota Stroke Association Annual Conference. www.braininjurymn.org

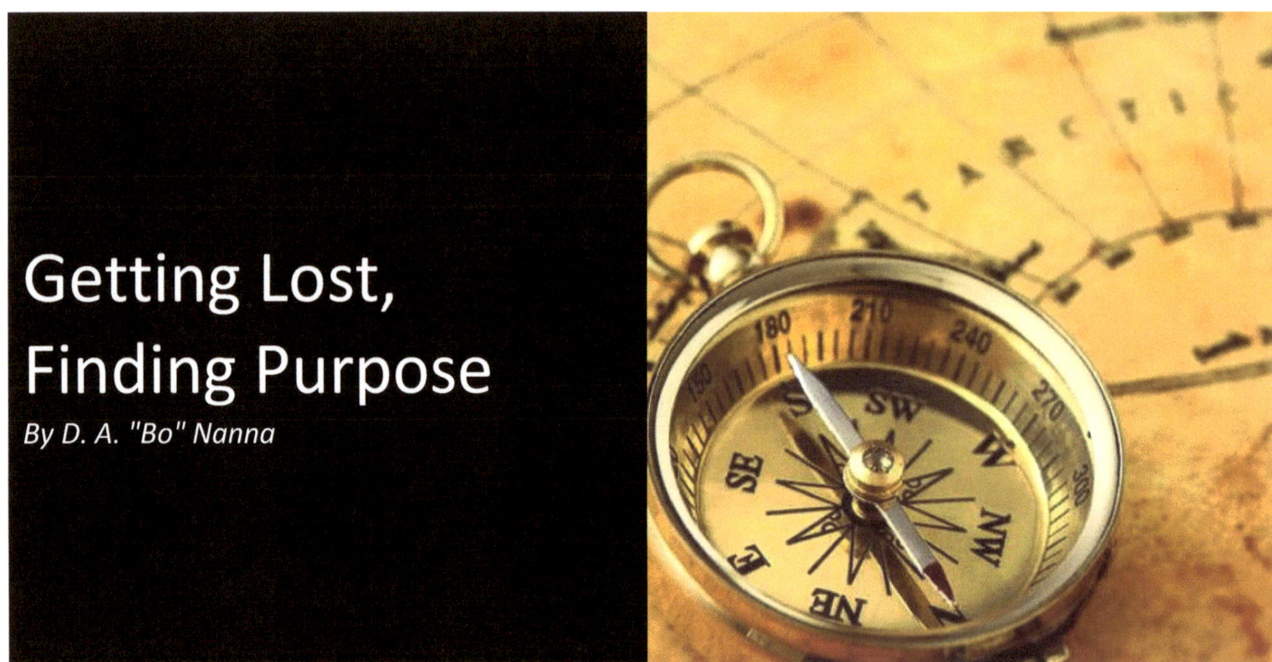

Getting Lost, Finding Purpose

By D. A. "Bo" Nanna

Eleven years ago, when my bike tire hit a crack in the road, it instantly stopped, but I didn't. I went flying over the handlebars and slid across the pavement until my head hit the curb. It caused plenty of road rash, a torn shoulder and a broken neck. Had I not been wearing a helmet, it might have been a lot worse.

Hours later, in the glare, noise and chaos of the emergency room, I remember doctors talking about a brain injury, but surely they didn't mean me. Three weeks later, when another doctor said my neck wouldn't need surgery, I badgered him into signing my return-to-work authorization.

As the abrasions and damaged vertebrae slowly improved, an excruciating headache persisted accompanied by a loud buzzing inside my skull. Exhausted and frustrated at work, I raged at my computer and shocked myself and others by yelling at my boss. Frequent talk-therapy got me through bad times, but a year later when things hadn't improved and another neurologist confirmed a brain injury, my wife and I asked what it meant. We both went blank when all he could offer was, "It is what it is."

"Four years later, after an array of antidepressants, seizure meds and alternative therapies, a new primary care physician suggested something called a brain injury support group."

Four years later, after an array of antidepressants, seizure meds and alternative therapies, a new primary care physician suggested something called a brain injury support group. I never considered myself someone who needed support, but my first meeting revealed how wrong I was, not just about the group, but about nearly everything else related to TBI. In this room full of people dealing with the

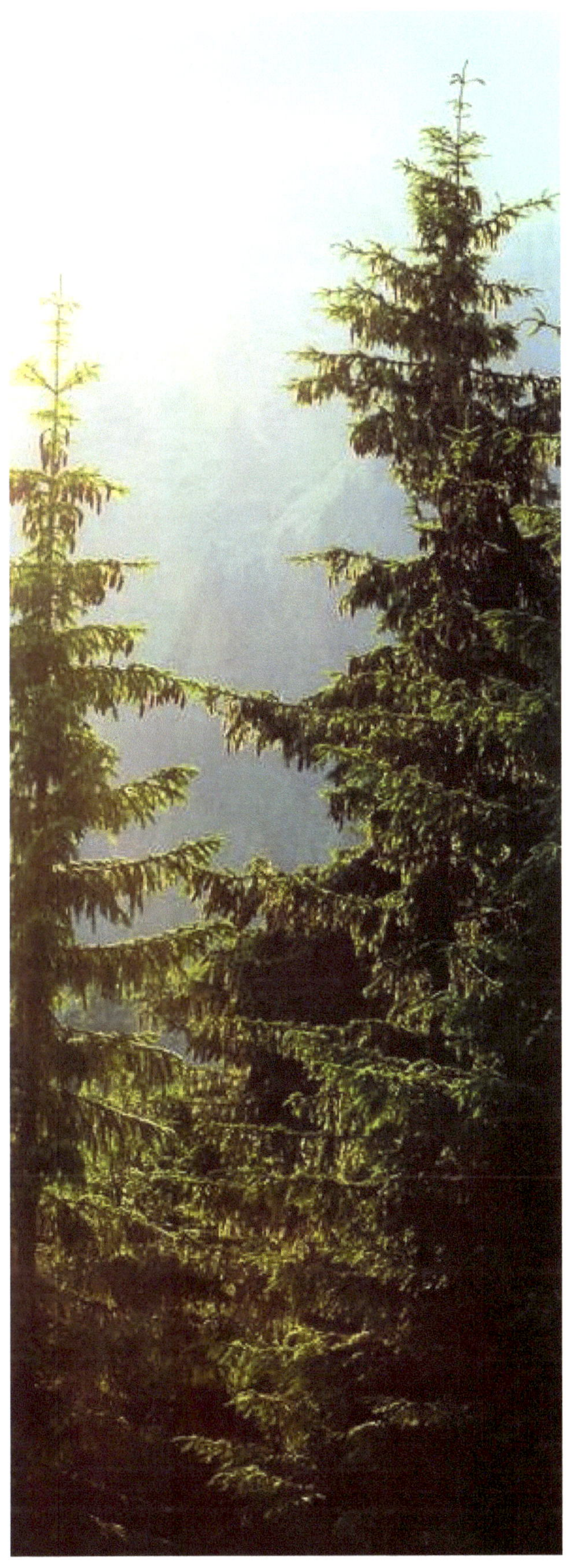

same issues I couldn't overcome, the tough Marine in me was reduced to tears of relief. I was not alone, and others wanted to help.

That first group meeting saved my life. When we moved back to Washington two years ago, the first thing I did was connect with a local group whose facilitator, Janice, is the most knowledgeable person I know when it comes to TBI and human behavior. For years she has selflessly helped others understand and live with brain change, encouraging each of us not just to survive, but to thrive in the best way possible.

A frequent theme of our group discussions is how to regain a sense of purpose in life after TBI. Most of us had family, work, relationships or special interests to feel meaningful and fulfilled, but brain injury often radically affects those anchors.

For me, not being able to work or do the physical things I enjoyed left tremendous emptiness. For better or worse, they were big parts of my identity. Hearing from other survivors of their similar challenges helped me recognize those missing elements and seek alternatives. Over the next few years I volunteered for a variety of things in non-profit organizations and a VA hospital.

In each situation, fulfillment didn't last, mostly because I reverted to my pre-TBI persona. I loved the purpose and people in each organization, wanted to contribute and accepted—even sought— greater responsibilities. But in short order, I let each one become time and energy obligations beyond my altered capabilities.

My noisy brain has difficulty listening and concentrating, but from every support group I try to bring home at least one "light bulb" epiphany. At one such meeting last year Janice's words about a purposeful life struck a resonant chord.

She knows we have dogs who, despite being recalcitrant terriers, comfort our home greatly. I told her about meeting a neighbor one day walking the dogs. He and his Labrador retriever are members of Kitsap County Search Dogs and we often talked about what they did. One day he asked if I'd like to join them to "get lost."

It turns out, regardless of the weather, they train every Saturday morning. In order to train search dogs, they need subjects, people for whom to search, and for that they always need volunteers.

So one Saturday my friend drove deep into a tree farm where we met the other teams. He briefed me about "Area Search" where the dog runs off-lead, sometimes at considerable distance from its handler. The dog finds a subject from the scent in the air then runs back to the handler and performs a trained response that says, "Hey, I found somebody!" The dog then brings its handler back to the subject to complete the find.

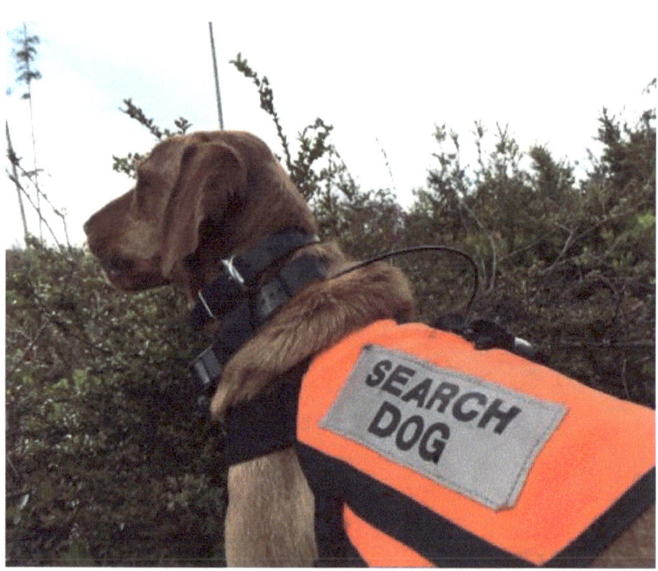

Phinny, K9 Partner of Handler "J.B." in Team 48.

"Trailing" dogs work nose-down, generally on a long-lead with their handler at the other end. From a scent sample, these dogs follow a trail to find a specific individual, even differentiating among multiple subjects.

On this day I was an air scent subject. I was issued a two-way radio then we hiked into the woods where my friend "placed" me and marked the location on GPS. Over the next two or three hours, handlers worked their dogs through various search scenarios finding multiple subjects, including me. The best part—when a dog successfully completes each find, it gets rewarded, usually with food, play or both, and I got to join the fun.

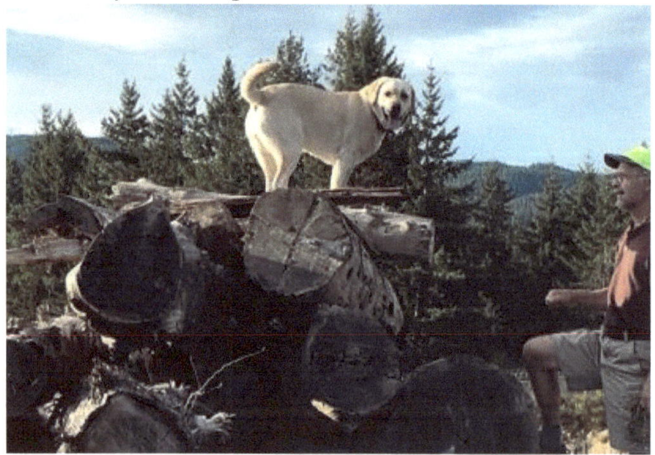

Tom & Sahale Training on Unstable Conditions

When I told Janice about volunteering to get lost, she smiled as I described sitting alone in the woods. It was quiet, although some areas are incredibly noisy from nearby highways, construction or air traffic. The only interruptions came when I heard the approaching bell of the well-trained dog, so proud to show its human partner what it had found. Then I witnessed the dog's unbridled joy celebrating its accomplishment. On top of that, everyone was grateful for me being there.

Janice knew immediately but it took a few more times for me to realize this could be my sense of purpose. In my first year of hiding I've made friends with retrievers, a bloodhound, three German and one Australian shepherd as well as a Belgian Malinois. I love the warm, sunny days and sitting alone in a pouring rain.

That eleven year-old headache and my "blender-brain" are still constant companions but seem less intrusive surrounded by nature and tall trees. I have to keep a list of the dogs, handlers and radio calls so I remember who's looking for me and when. Sometimes I want to get more involved, but I remind myself it's not possible—or even necessary—for me to do more than sit under a tree and smell like a human to contribute to their rigorous training.

Now I spend most Saturday mornings as a target of amazing partnerships between smart canines and dedicated humans as they hone team skills for potentially life-saving missions. Each dog is unique, but they all want nothing more than to make that successful find to fulfill their purpose. I just needed to get lost in order to find mine.

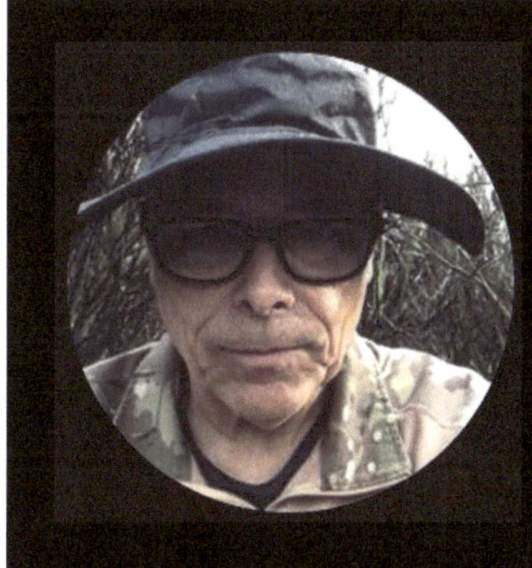

Meet D. A. "Bo" Nanna

Bo survived a 2008 brain injury from a bicycling accident. His career included marketing and management in pharmaceutical, biotech and non-profit healthcare although he remains forever a "no longer active-duty Marine."

His LinkedIn profile, if he had one, would read: "Personal assistant for two Scottish Terriers; excels at poop collection and disposal. Enjoys spending time outdoors playing hide and seek with canines."

Living With Hope

By Patrick Brigham

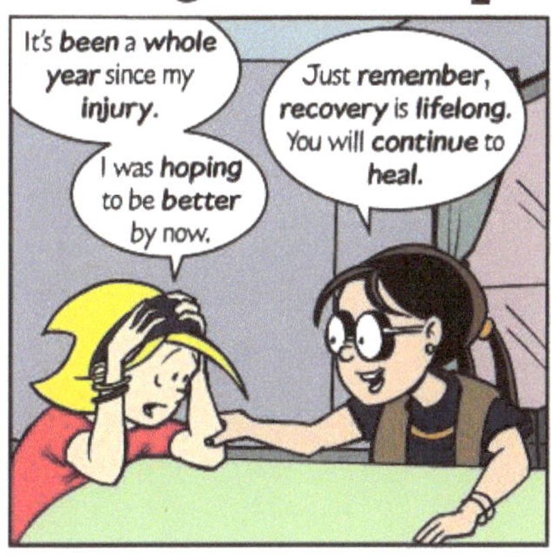

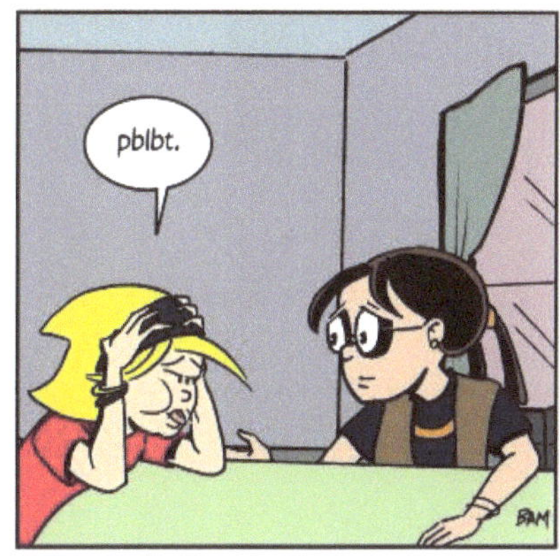

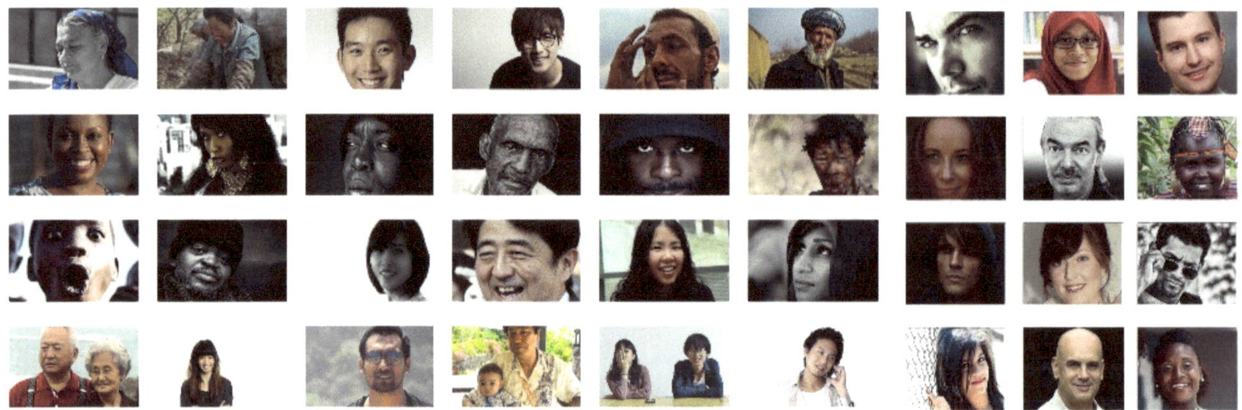

In Less Time Than it Took You to Read this, Someone New Sustained a Brain Injury.

In Less Time Than it Took You to Read this, Someone New Sustained a Brain Injury.

In Less Time Than it Took You to Read this, Someone New Sustained a Brain Injury.

In Less Time Than it Took You to Read this, Someone New Sustained a Brain Injury.

In Less Time Than it Took You to Read this, Someone New Sustained a Brain Injury.

It's Time to End the Silence.

www.tbihopeandinspiration.com

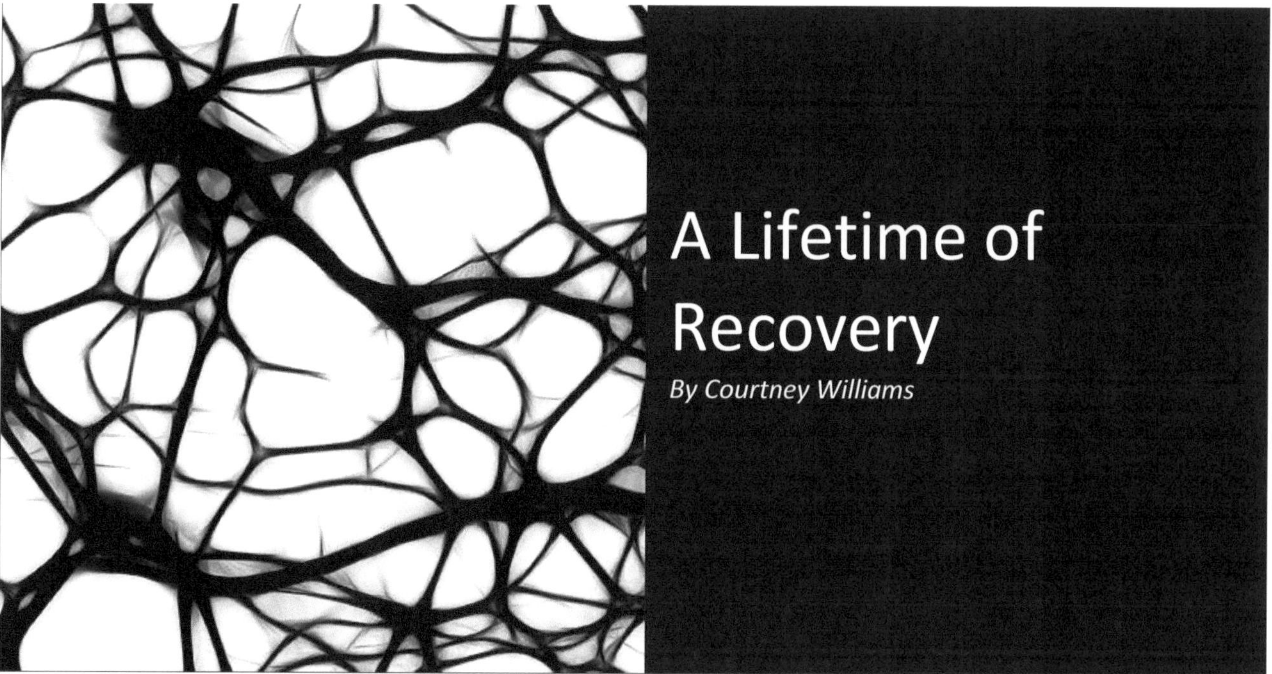

Flash back to three years to this day, when doctors told me that I had bleeding in my brain and what they referred to as a Traumatic Brain Injury. They ran through a list of many things they said I may experience or may or may not be able to do again. This ranged from nausea, loss/excess thirst, loss of taste, extreme fatigue, debilitating migraines, short and long term memory loss, poor attention/concentration, slow processing speed, dizziness, poor balance and sleep disturbances.

They said I could experience feelings of confusion, depression, anxiety, sudden mood changes, and irritability. All of which are common and that often occur as a result of brain damage, but something no one ever told me or my family that I would also go through a period of what I call "grieving my old self." To this day, I still can't remember exactly who I was before my accident, and that's a kind of hurt I wouldn't wish on anyone.

> *"To this day, I still can't remember exactly who I was before my accident, and that's a kind of hurt I wouldn't wish on anyone."*

Imagine waking up one day in a body that looks like you, but you know it isn't. Your life externally seems the same, but everything on the inside has changed. Simple tasks that were once mindless to do are now completely exhausting. Every single thing you try to do, just as you did before is now nearly impossible. Even when you know what you want to say, for some reason you cannot find the words.

When I was going through the worst of it, I didn't know how to tell others what I was experiencing. During one of these attempts to communicate with a friend, is when I knew something had changed, I was different. I'll always feel that a little part of me died that day as well. This isn't just a little cold that you take medicine for and you're cured, TBIs are a lifetime injury.

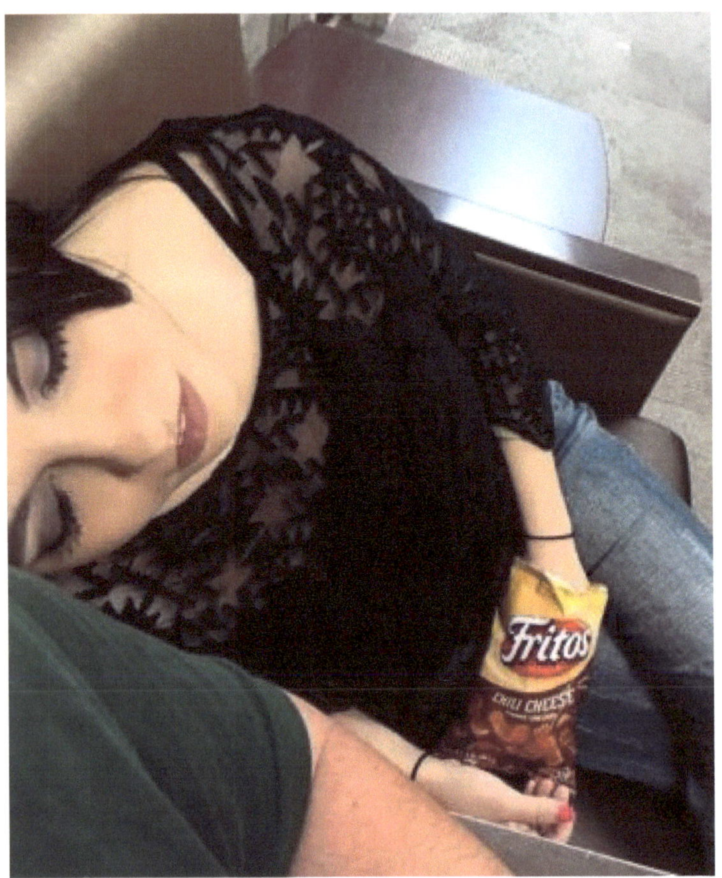

Falling Asleep Eating Chips

I denied my shortcomings for a long time, probably about a year. I wanted so desperately to do all the things I used to do, but by staying in denial, it made things worse for me instead. It would send me from setback to setback, lasting for days or even weeks at a time. The emotional exhaustion was unreal, and the pain in my head was nothing like I had ever experienced before.

Anytime I ever felt even a tiniest bit of energy, I would jump back up only to run myself to the ground again. I kept thinking, "I can do this. I just have to push through. I can beat this and be better. Having a brain injury is not going to change me. This won't stop me from living my life and doing all the things I used to and want to do."

Wrong again! After months, I was finally placed in a brain rehabilitation center where I learned that you can't just "push through" these things. You have to show your brain again how things work and are used. That is around the time when things got even harder for me. I became more depressed, longing for what I used to be and seeing how far from that I was.

Since no one explained these constant emotional ups and downs, to my family and friends, they would just look at me and say I was the same, and nothing's changed so I needed to stop worrying. They would even say things like, "oh, you can't even tell you've been in an accident!" Knowing they had good intentions and they just didn't understand, I turned inward more, because I couldn't show them how much about me had actually changed, how lost and hopeless I was feeling. These are emotions that you wouldn't know someone is feeling just looking at them. I never felt more alone and misunderstood in my life, and it made the grieving process so much harder than it had to be.

It still surprises me after seeing so many doctors that none even mentioned the possibility that I may experience the grief of losing "myself," the person I was before the accident. If I would have known that then, I could have tried to educate myself more to help my loved ones understand, and then maybe I wouldn't have been so self-isolating, making a bad situation, even worse.

It wasn't until I took the time for self-reflection, which came after two years of living my "new life", that I let go of all that I had been ignoring because it was too hard to believe my life had changed that suddenly. I finally accepted what had happened to me and my body, and I'll never stop trying to get back to "normal", but it was time to accept that this is me now. That's also the moment when I was able to really start healing through the emotional trauma of the past two years. Most importantly, it allowed me to truly connect with myself internally and become more spiritual. I figured out that even though I may operate differently now with some limitations, I'm still me. There is still light shining here. There is still breath in my lungs, and the sun shines on my face.

And while I may not always completely recognize the person behind my eyes the way I used to, I'm much closer to understanding her than I was yesterday. It just gave me the perfect opportunity for a fresh start and new chances. To anyone else struggling like I was, please have faith, because I'm living proof that there is hope, and anyone can rise above their challenges and spread their sunshine!

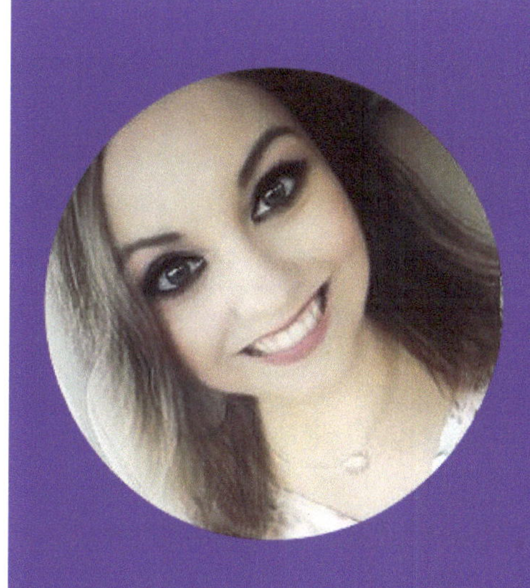

Meet Courtney Williams

Courtney is a thirty-two year old Baton Rouge native who sustained her TBI as a result of a horrific car accident. She was resuscitated, intubated, and placed on a ventilator upon admission to the hospital. Before her injury she worked in the medical field and was in school for nursing as helping those who cannot help themselves has always been her passion. She hopes to finish nursing school in the near future. In her free time, she enjoys spending time with her three babies: Rennie, Kendall, and Erica. Dogs are also a passion of hers and early in her career she became the Managing Editor of a national dog magazine. She hopes to inspire and mentor others by sharing her story and has recently started a blog.

Let's Get Social!

What do over 30,000 people from 26 countries and five continents all have in common? They are all members of our vibrant Facebook family at /TBIHopeandInspiration

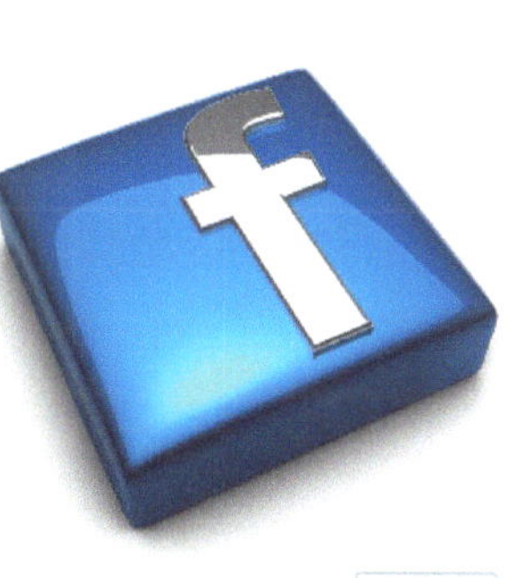

Join our Facebook Family Today!

Learning Curves

By Rebecca Veenstra

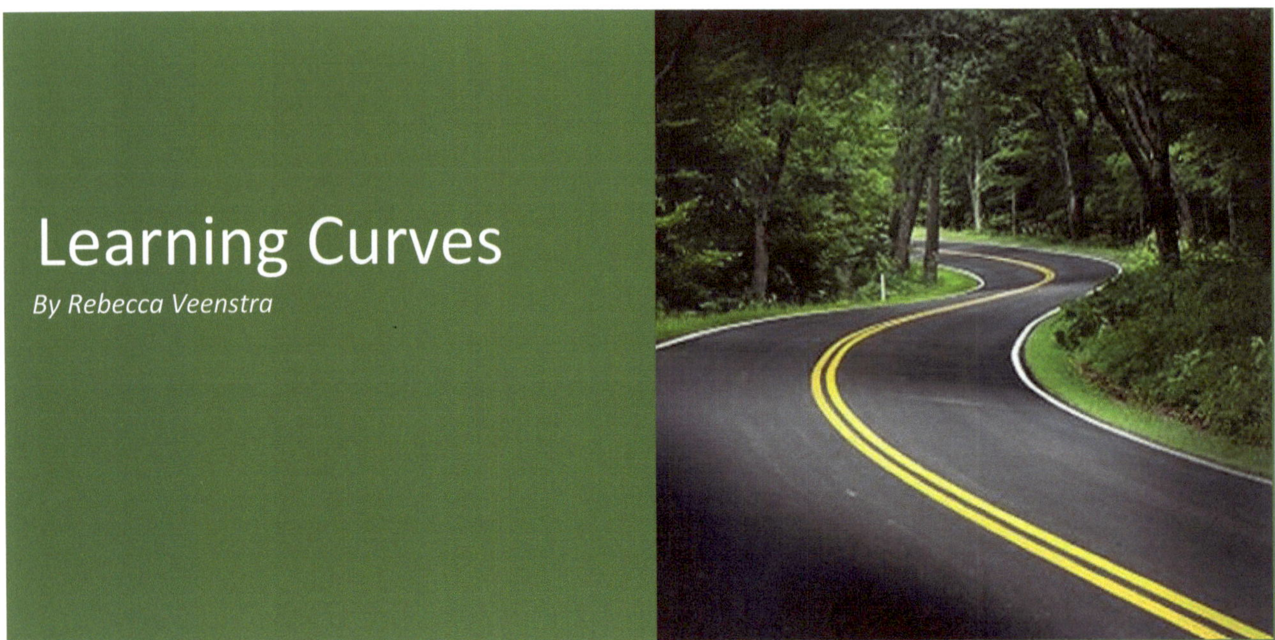

In 2014 on my way to work one morning a dump truck pulled in front of me. I remember little else besides slamming on my brakes and screaming "No!" The aftermath was grueling with surgeries, wheelchairs and a lovely plastic brace. Despite its being custom molded to my body, I got sick of trying to hide it under my clothes.

With that contraption outside of my clothing while in my wheelchair with my left arm in a cast and my torn up face, I was a sight to behold. Eventually my spine fracture healed. I received a new titanium hip to replace the one that died from avascular necrosis, a vocabulary word you don't hear every day. The doctors took almost two years to diagnose the crippling nerve pain. Now at least I know what causes the fiery stabbing in my thigh. I have graduated from a four-wheel walker that I nick named my "man-magnet" to a very snappy platform cane—the accessory every middle-aged woman longs for.

"She incorrectly deemed that whatever head injury I had sustained was completely resolved. This was based on my ability to draw a clock."

Even after colliding with a dump truck, I was never evaluated at the Emergency Room for a head injury. After I'd been in the nursing home for about a month, they had to release me. A few days before they sent me on my way, I received a very brief visit from a woman that was trained to evaluate dementia patients for basic orientation. She incorrectly deemed that whatever head injury I had sustained was completely resolved. This was based on my ability to draw a clock. I should also mention that the room she met me in was my hospital room; where—during the evaluation, I was facing and looking at the clock on the wall.

During the month I was in the hospital I spent to first two-and-a-half weeks vomiting and lost forty pounds. I was eventually released from the nursing home. It was six months before they realized my thigh bone was dying.

During this time no one made any mention of TBI. I mixed my words up constantly, floated around in a blank mind, missing appointments and felt a sense of disorientation that only a fellow TBI patient can fully appreciate. It was over a year after the crash that I got sent for a neuropsych exam. I am a smart woman and went into that test thinking that I would do well on the test - until I learned it was an eight-hour test. I admit that that I was a little intimidated.

Fast-forward about ten minutes into the test as I sat baffled trying to understand why the simple task the doctor has asked me to perform seemed completely impossible. Two full years later the insurance company sent me for an Independent Medical Evaluation (IME). If you are not familiar with an IME, you are fortunate. I was driven for four hours in crazy traffic by a driver selected by the insurance company to the testing location.

Four hours into the eight-hour test I crumbled into tears and fell asleep on the examiners table. Needless to say, they rescheduled the last part of the test for another day. I was driven a second four hours to complete the test. The driver nearly collided with another vehicle. I screamed so loudly I almost lost my voice. Suffice to say, I bombed the test. The IME doctor explained this away by saying I needed a medication review and by actually mocking my attempts to explain what it was like living with a TBI.

As if there weren't enough reports on my poor brain, another IME was assigned to me by the defense attorney for the guy who nearly killed me. Thankfully though, my neuropsychologist stood by me, comforted me, and most importantly explained and assisted me with the many mind-boggling symptoms a person with TBI and PTSD juggles every day.

I have real deficits that include light sensitivity, constant tinnitus, auditory sensitivity, and neuro-fatigue. I often read articles in this magazine that I feel I could have written on that subject. My favorite description is a woman who wrote it was a "Non-negotiable exhaustion." There are days that my phone can be four feet away and I cannot muster up the strength to move to get it. I've sat in complete silence for entire afternoons listening to my ears ring feeling not a single shred of energy to do a thing.

> **I was sent to cognitive therapy where I slowly learned to accept my new deficits.**

I was sent to cognitive therapy where I slowly learned to accept my new deficits. More importantly, I learned ways to compensate for them. I really thought I would just wake up one day and all these symptoms would just go away - like the flu or a cold. I didn't apply myself and I did not accept the diagnosis. Day after day it continued to haunt me with a cruel vengeance. I would often find myself in situations where I had no idea would trigger me and sap every ounce of energy I had.

To this day, after a staggering amount of cognitive therapy, pelvic floor therapy, physical therapy, psychotherapy, EMDR therapy, nerve blocks, surgeries, and physical training I find myself blindsided by my deficits. You would think there would be predictability or consistency to such things, but really there isn't. I can strategize and insulate myself, but as soon as I stray from my cozy cocoon of a house and venture into the world, there is no question that my TBI and my PTSD will affect the way I experience everything.

Five years later and everything has changed. The old me is a distant shadow that I can barely conjure up. The constant disoriented feeling persists, but I can better define my new self to some degree and speak relatively intelligently - as long as I'm not being flooded. I might not remember any of it tomorrow, but they say to live in the moment. Today my life is a succession of moments – some painful, some enjoyable, but it's my life, and I'm doing the best I can.

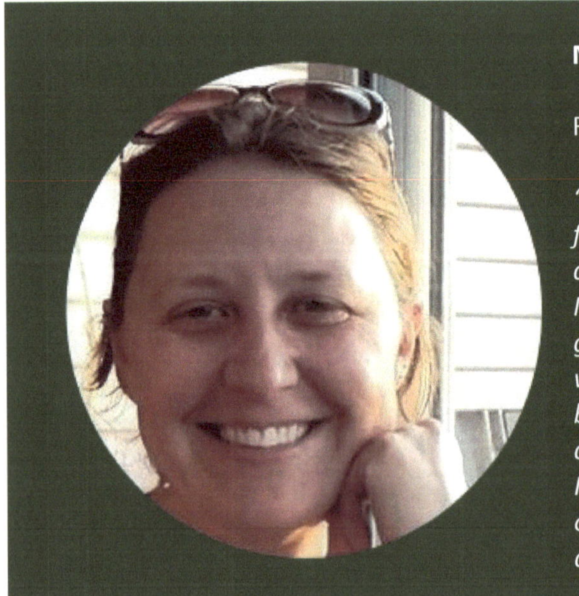

Meet Rebecca Veenstra

Rebecca writes…

"I am 47 years old. I was an herbalist, runner, work out fanatic, health food nut and writer before a run in with a dump truck in 2014 changed my life forever. I live in Northern Michigan with my two Chihuahuas. I enjoy gardening and photography. This is my first piece of writing since the crash. It feels good to have my words back again. I am beginning to think of ways I can pay back all the kindness and caring I received through my recovery. I hope to someday find a path that gives me the opportunity to advocate for and support others with TBI and PTSD."

Contributors Wanted

Share Your Story in HOPE Magazine

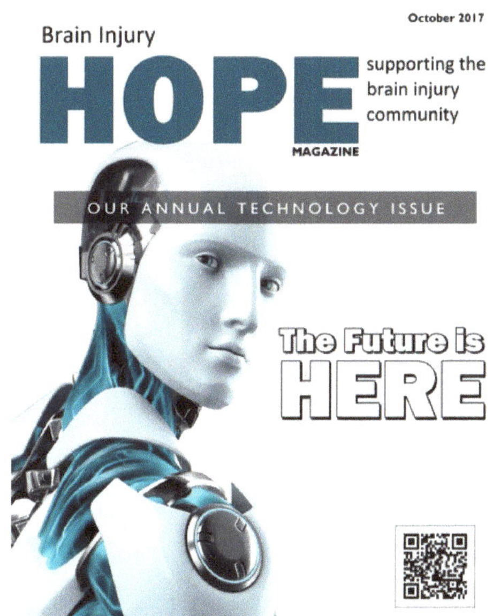

Do you have a story that you'd like to share with the world? If so, we'd love to hear from you! HOPE Magazine is always looking for stories to publish in our monthly magazine.

It doesn't matter whether you are a survivor, caregiver, family member or part of the professional or support community. We ALL have something to offer!

Your Story Has Value

► We prefer an article length of 800-1,000 words. Longer or shorter pieces will be considered.

► When submitting, please include a photo or photos to be included with your piece.

► We happily offer a link back to your blog, website, or most anywhere pertinent.

► Please include a short biography, preferably under 150 words.

► Please include 2-3 photos to accompany your submission

► Previously published pieces are acceptable for submission. Just let us know where your piece was previously published.

► Any topic that resonates within the brain injury/concussion community will be considered.

► Submissions that directly or indirectly promote a specific product, or business will be rejected.

► Submissions need to either be in Microsoft Word or in Notepad format. PDF's and links to content posted on an existing website will not be considered for publication.

Submission is Easy. Email Your Story to: mystory@tbihopeandinspiration.com

Caregiver Anger

By Lynn Kaye

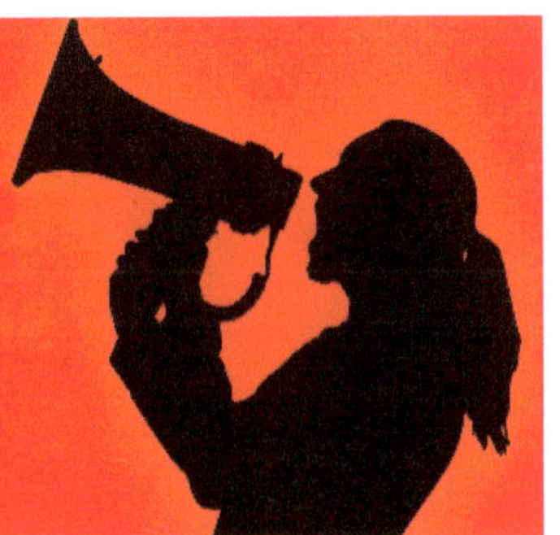

I have been a caregiver for my husband for eight years.

We have been married for twenty-six years.

Sometimes I am sad, but now I am mostly angry...

Angry that we were fairly young when he became ill. He was 53 and I was 44. Angry that the last two years of my mother's life were focused on caring for him instead of her. Angry that I didn't get to spend more time with her.

Angry that my best income earning years have been taken from me. Angry that we will have less money to live on since I had to retire early and become a caregiver. Angry that I am now responsible for keeping us financially stable for much longer than most retired people. Angry that every decision I make revolves around how it affects him.

Angry that I must walk on eggshells to avoid catastrophic reactions from him. Angry that I have to choose to put him on medications with horrendous side effects and be the only one to weigh benefits versus risks. Angry that my spouse is now visually impaired and how that affects every single thing. Angry that I have to spend my time researching the best medications, foods, vitamins, activities, alternative therapies, insurance plans and strategies for daily living.

Angry that I have to find the funds to pay for what he needs. Angry that I am too exhausted to do much self-care. Angry that we can't have a normal back and forth conversation. Angry that he believes I am the reason for our communication issues. Angry that no one really cares what we are going through. Angry that we live in slow motion.

Angry that I spend a massive amount of time waiting. Angry that he has no concept of time so it is up to me to figure out how long it will take him to get ready. Angry that every day may take a different amount of time to get ready depending on how tired he is. Angry that he has no patience for waiting no matter where we are, so I have to bring something to occupy him just in case.

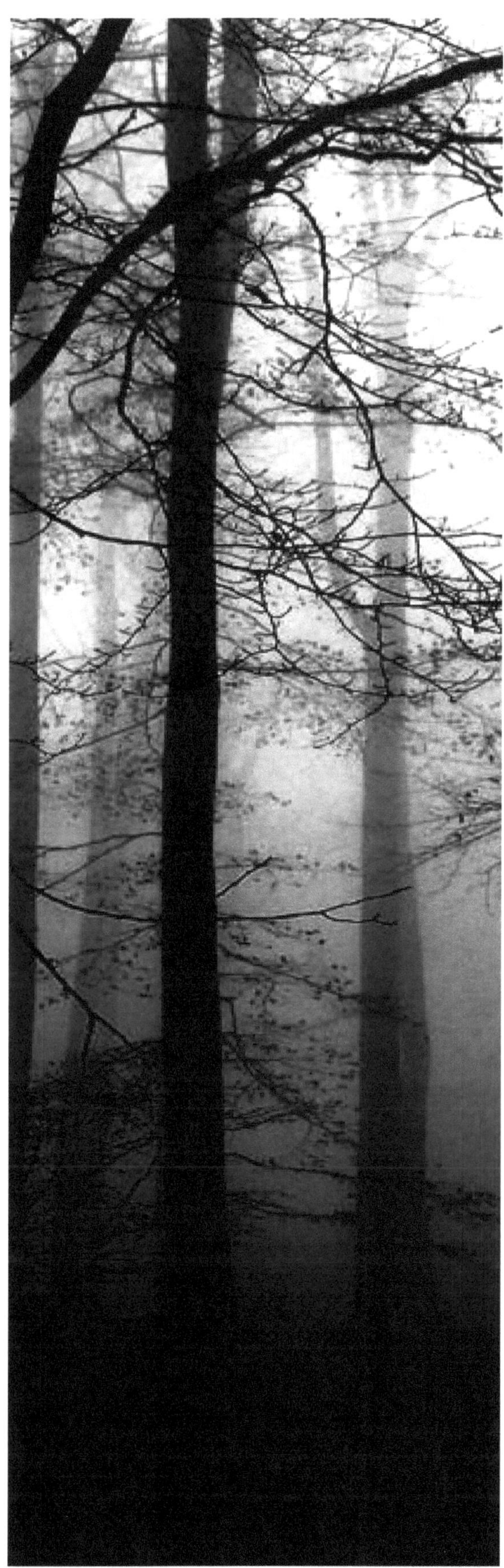

Angry that if I go away, I get nasty phone calls if I am gone too long. Angry when he says that I am no fun when everything I do revolves around helping him having fun.

Angry that I've lost the motivation to improve my situation. Angry that I can't take overnight trips with my daughter anymore. Angry that it is up to me to make sure he gets some kind of exercise every day. Angry that I am losing empathy. Angry that I allow aggressive behavior towards me because I have no choice. Angry that no one visits. Angry that no one knows how hard this is.

Angry that we appear to be such a cute couple in public. Angry that once we are alone, he becomes Mr. Nasty. Angry that he has no friends. Angry that some family can't handle the new him. Angry that it seems I will never get a break as he won't allow anyone but me to help him. Angry that I must resort to therapeutic lying to keep peace.

Angry that I have to prepare for the future without knowing what it may be. Angry that almost every interaction with him becomes an argument. Angry that he seems like a child most of the time. Angry that I am never alone in my own home. Angry that no one asks to take him out once in a while. Angry that I feel guilty going anywhere since he can't.

Angry that I can't show the slightest negative emotion because he will mirror it and it is exaggerated. Angry that I am completely depended on by someone who can be very mean. Angry that he is unaware and believes I am the one "losing it." Angry that it takes so long for him to do anything. Angry that most of the tasks he can do I have to do over, but I don't let him know that.

Angry that he blames me for everything. Angry that I have to be the boss. Angry that I have to pick my battles. Angry that we can't be spontaneous. Angry that I thought he should have a service dog, but I end up doing all the work taking care of her. Angry that traveling is very challenging.

Angry that I have to be prepared and remember everything. Angry that thinking for two is exhausting. Angry that he can be embarrassing in public. Angry that each year I'm starting to notice regression. Angry that he has no reasoning skills. Angry that life is so hard.

Angry that I no longer have an equal partner. Angry that I must put on a happy face, be encouraging and celebrate small wins every day.

Angry that I can't just walk away. Angry that he says he wishes he were dead every day. Angry that no matter what I try it doesn't make him content. Angry that I have to drive us everywhere forever while he complains. Angry that going places isn't fun. Angry that I can't leave anything in a spot that it doesn't belong. Everything has its place for him.

Angry that watching him struggle to eat with visual impairment and one hand is still hard. Angry that I have to keep track of everything. Angry that all the household chores and maintenance are my job. Angry that he makes messes and I have to clean them up. Angry that he wants to spend all his money. Angry that he doesn't listen to me, causing unsafe situations. Angry that when he is tired, he gets mad and wants a divorce even though his is incapable of caring for himself.

Angry that in front of others he is on his best behavior. Angry that I didn't set aside weekly time for myself right away. Angry that I am angry, and it is a waste of my time and energy. Angry that I already feel old at fifty-two.

Most of all, I am angry that I care too much to give up.

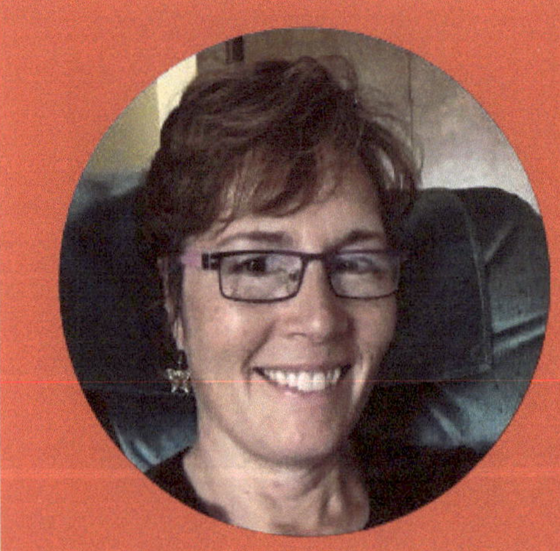

Meet Lynn Kaye

Lynn Kaye lives near Chicago with her husband and his Service Dog. She enjoys walking around the neighborhood, coffee and coloring. She spends a lot of time reading about brain injury and learning strategies from caregivers and survivors.

Ignoring the Inner Voice

By David A. Grant

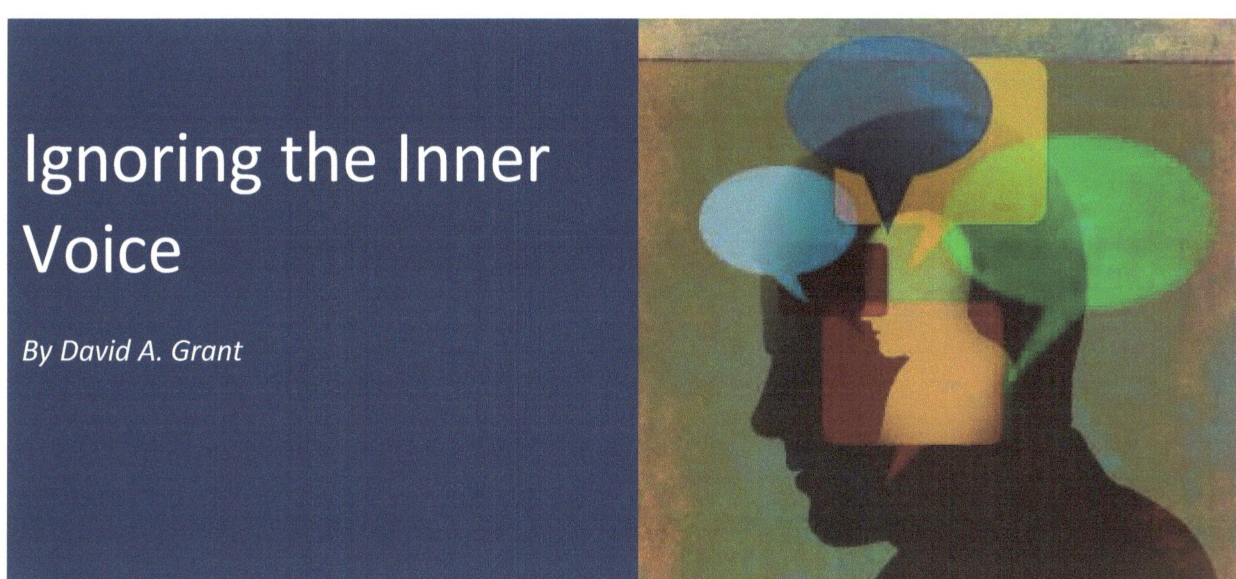

Next month will mark the nine year anniversary of my brain injury. It was on a chilly November day in southern New Hampshire that my life, and the lives of all those close to me, changed forever. I was run over by a teenage, newly-licensed driver - struck down while I was cycling.

My broken bones, bruises, and lacerations from the shattered windshield are now all distant memories, but my brain injury lingers on. Unlike my broken arm that had a date-stamp for recovery, my TBI will be with me for the duration. For as long as I have a heartbeat, I will continue to recover.

Over the last few years, my gains have exceeded what members of the medical community predicted as my outcome. I am back to work on a full-time basis, helping to support our household in a meaningful way. If you were to meet me today, providing it wasn't a bad TBI day, you would never know that I faced near death and live with a hidden disability.

> *"If you were to meet me today, providing it wasn't a bad TBI day, you would never know that I faced near death and live with a hidden disability."*

Dare I say that life is reasonably normal these days? I still have "TBI stuff." On a bad day, when exhaustion kicks in, my brain injury symptoms come back with a vengeance. Hide 'n seek with words is a common outcome. Though my word-finding challenges are far less than they were before, they still resurface at unexpected times. These days I shrug it off. It goes with the TBI territory.

Recently, I was reminded in an unexpected way how tough things really were early on. A new friend and I were having a conversation when he uttered a jaw-dropping line.

"I was introduced to you back in 2011. When you spoke to me, it was nothing but gibberish," he said, much to my surprise. "Someone pulled me aside and told me that you had a bad head injury."

Here's where it gets interesting. Did I use this as a point on the linear timeline to feel good about how far I've come? About how infrequently I now have audible speech challenges? Did I quietly pat myself on the back, congratulating myself on my ongoing recovery?

Not even close!

In a single tick of the clock, I felt humiliated. I was embarrassed at my behavior from so many years ago. In an instant, I felt "less than" my friend. I immediately felt sub-human. My self-worth plummeted, and though I can't say for certain, my shoulders probably slumped. I was completely deflated.

And then the voices started. Not out loud, mind you. That would be more of a psychotic episode. Rather, I am referencing that inner narrative that we all have, brain-injured or not.

"He knows that you are disabled and pities you."
"What an idiot I am. I must have looked like a complete fool."
"If someone told him that I had a head injury, that means that lots of people were talking about me. I bet none of it was good."

And the toughest of all, *"You are never going to be normal again. You will spend the rest of your life never living up to the standards of those uninjured. You will ALWAYS be 'less than.'"*

As much as I would like to say that this was a one-off event, it's not. In the quiet of home, when something TBI related comes up, I am indeed able to shrug it off.

But when I'm out and about, in public with other people, and TBI symptoms resurface, it's a whole different scenario.

So, what is the solution? The first step is awareness. You can't change behavior that you are blind to. Though painful, just being aware that the inner narrative is false is a great place to start. But awareness alone means that no changes have been made. While I can't help what I think, I do have the power to respond to my thoughts.

While I don't do this audibly, I can take mental control of things and remind myself that I am a miracle. If I believed the medical professionals, I wasn't supposed to have the life I have today. I am an equal member of the human family – no better or no worse than anyone else. And I sometimes need to remind myself that I am not alone in having an invisible disability.

> # While I can't help what I think, I do have the power to respond to my thoughts.

As I move through my day-to-day life, I pass by others with hidden challenges. That cashier at the market might have fibromyalgia. The person that I just held the door for may be living with depression. The list goes on. Many of us have heard the old saying, "Be kind to people as everyone is fighting their own battle."

I have a heartbeat; therefore, I have challenges. You have a heartbeat, and it is a near certainty that you have challenges too. If I look at the fact that we all share challenges, then I'm less alone, and simply an average member of the human family. I belong here. And isn't that all that we really want - just to belong?

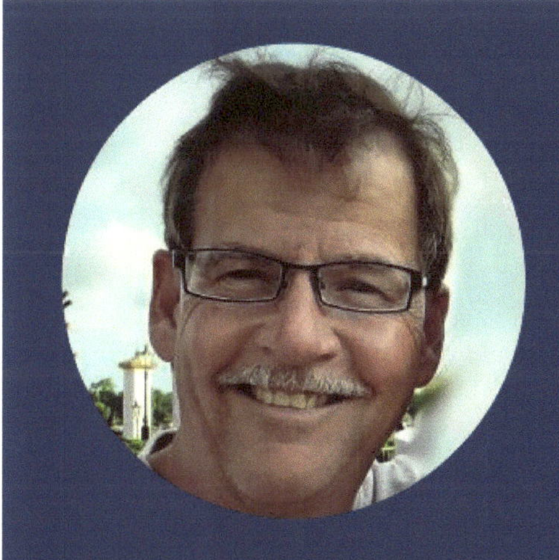

Meet David A. Grant

David A. Grant is a freelance writer based out of southern New Hampshire and the publisher of HOPE Magazine. He is the author of Metamorphosis, Surviving Brain Injury.

He is also a contributing author to Chicken Soup for the Soul, Recovering from Traumatic Brain Injuries. David is a BIANH Board Member. David is a regular contributing writer to Brainline.org, a PBS sponsored website.

THE TRUTH ABOUT
CONCUSSION

A concussion is a mild traumatic brain injury (mTBI).
Most concussions occur without losing consciousness.

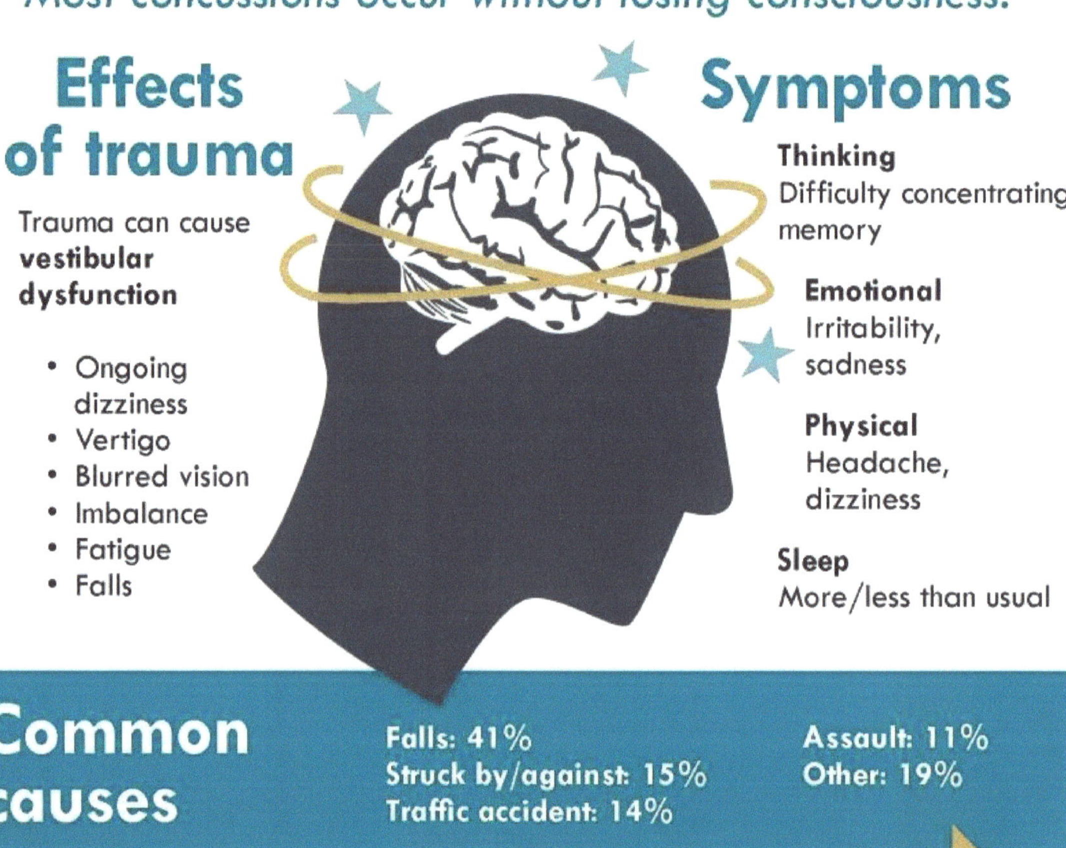

Know the Signs - Get Medical Attention

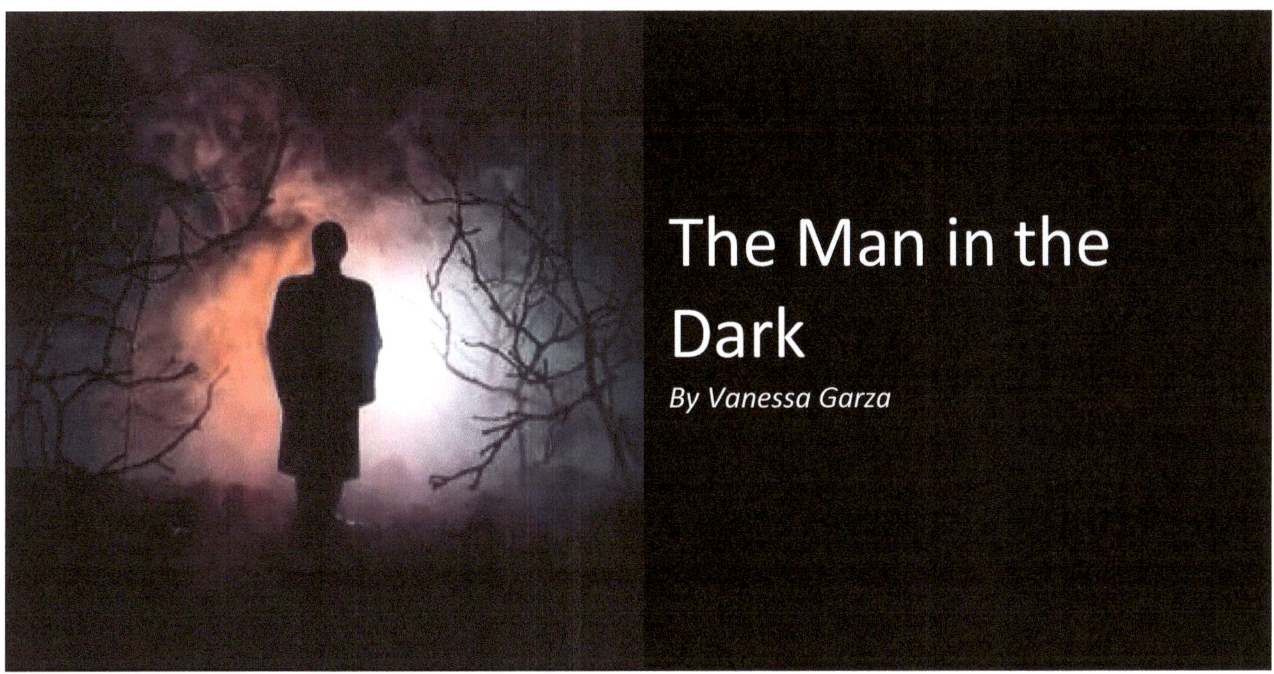

"Can you talk?" I typed anxiously. "I'm confused and want to talk to someone who's been through this before."

I lay awake next to my sleeping husband while record-breaking snow accumulated on our lawn. From the exterior, my house resembled others on my street - 1920's colonials, sparkling with fresh snow, filled with families snuggled in warm beds. From the interior, a different scene unfolded. I had met someone online. I was engulfed in a chat with a stranger, on my computer, under the covers, in the dark, in the middle of the night.

As my lips tingled and chest tightened, I heard snow plows rumble outside. I felt the hot breath of my 75-pound dog sleep-panting at my feet. And the smell. It was the familiar scent of my husband's crusty white t-shirt. I breathed forcefully to prevent a panic attack, but the blizzard inside me raged stronger than the white flurries dancing outside on that wintry night.

"Our conversation took place on a Facebook page. It was not a dating site, a cheating page, or a page to meet people, single or married."

I could feel tears running down my cheeks. I don't remember if I was audibly sobbing, but my heart broke. This man. His words. I couldn't believe it. He didn't know, and I didn't know, but he was about to change my life.

Our conversation took place on a Facebook page. It was not a dating site, a cheating page, or a page to meet people, single or married. The site was an online support group for anyone impacted by brain Arteriovenous Malformations (AVMs), an affliction that had consumed my life over the prior year.

I was 36-years old. I had it all - a devoted husband, two healthy children, a career, a red brick home, even the quintessential yellow Labrador frolicking in fresh snow. I also had a malformation in my brain, a tangle of blood vessels that could burst, cause a stroke, and kill me.

Leading up to that conversation in the dark, I had met with a dozen neurosurgeons on the East Coast. The doctors said my condition was rare, that I could not be fixed, that I should not be fixed. "There are too many risks," they said. "If you elect brain surgery, you could end up blind, among other unpredictable deficits, including a brain bleed in the operating room. It's likely that you'll go into surgery with 100 percent of your senses, but awake with some missing."

They told me I had to live with, but try to ignore, my ticking time-bomb. Doctors treating AVMs often suggest a watch and wait approach, due to the rarity and complexity of these congenital defects.

Except one doctor in the Southwest, who said he could safely remove the web in my brain. He said it with confidence, with gusto. How I wanted to hear those words, I think. But fixing me would require surgery, several of them, the longest lasting twelve hours. First, he would inject glue into my brain, then rip open my head, crack open my skull, resect a piece of my brain, secure it with plates and screws, and staple it back together, a couple of times. But every step risked a stroke in the operating room and chance of death on the table.

I initially assumed early detection of my AVM was a blessing, until I realized it was a curse. I faced an incomprehensible decision: to elect multiple complicated brain surgeries against the advice of all but one doctor, or to gamble that my brain would never explode in my lifetime.

I viewed both scenarios as equally devastating. Either cracking my head open from the outside on purpose, or from the inside on its own terms, could kill me or leave me disabled. Every direction I looked pointed to signs of death, blindness, paralysis, memory loss, stroke.

I spent sleepless nights on this Facebook page. Previously, I had met a mom whose young daughter suffered an AVM hemorrhage. She did not escape unscathed; she suffered paralysis and is destined for a lifetime of therapy to regain

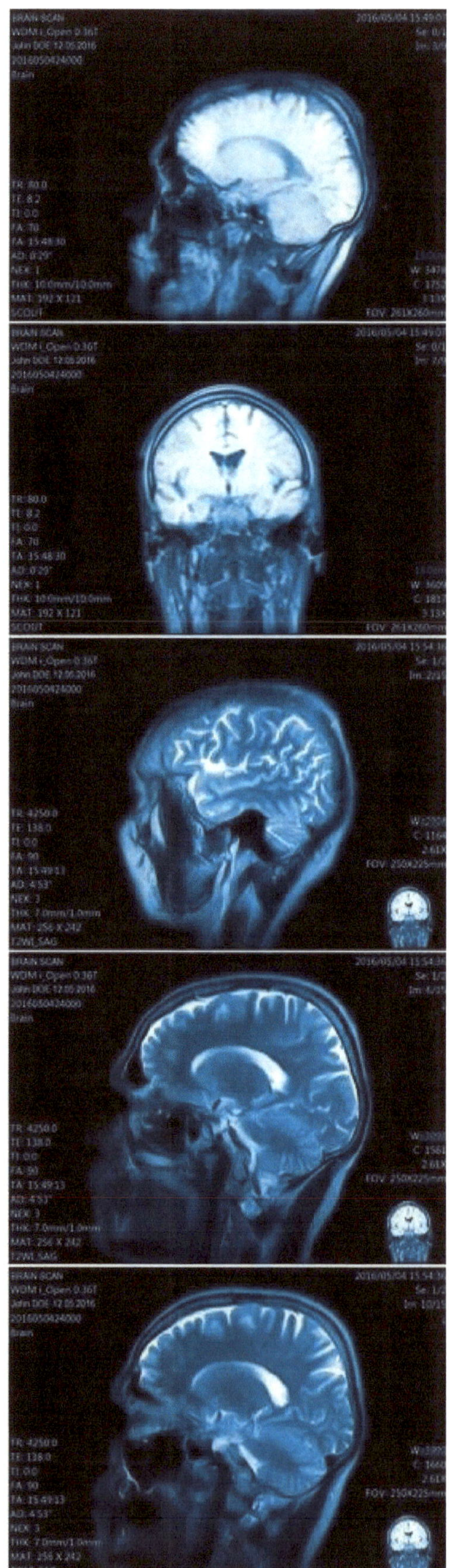

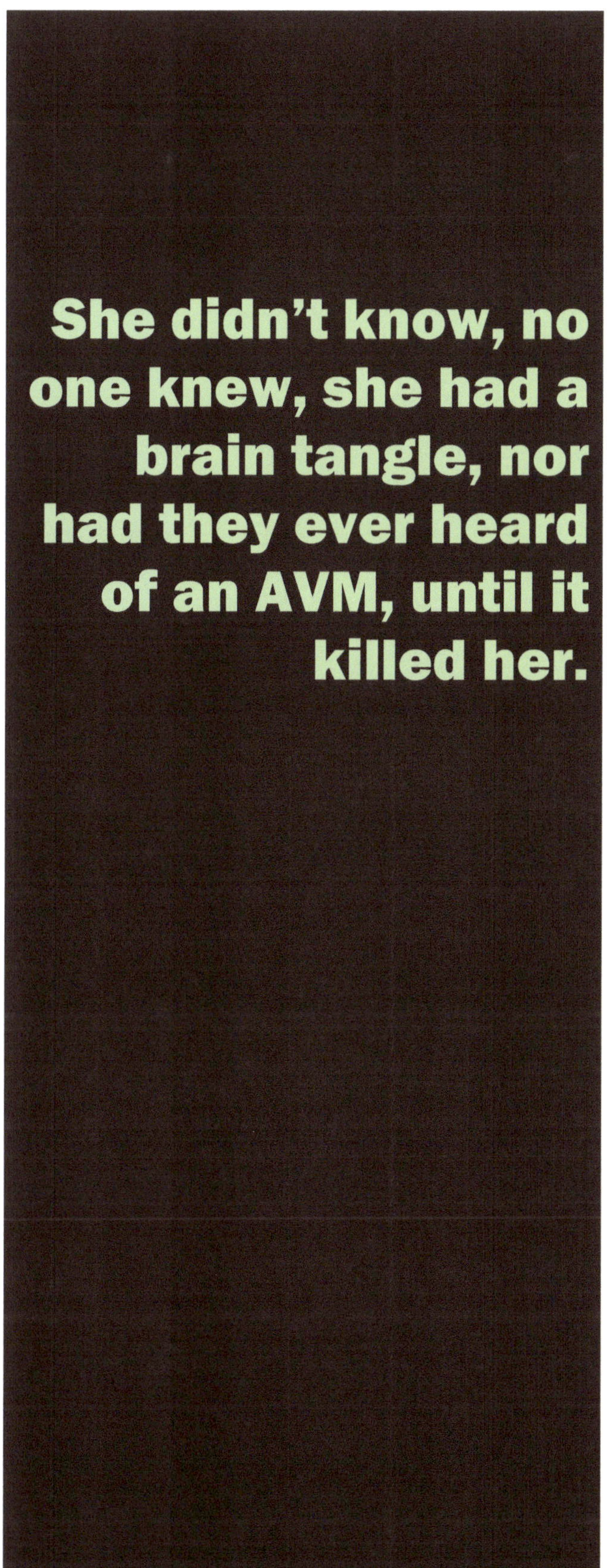

skills like feeding herself and tying her shoes. I hoped this mom was awake that night. I needed to talk to someone, anyone who knew about brain AVMs.

But then I found a different man online. I asked directly, "I have seen many doctors about my AVM. Most of them say it is too dangerous to remove, but one doctor says he can do it. Do you have any advice?"

I shivered under the blankets. I didn't know this man, but I was desperate for advice. My heart nearly barreled out of my chest.

"Please, if you have the chance, remove that beast," he wrote. "It is a killer."

I stared at the screen feeling like my eyes might pop out of their sockets. I did not expect his adamant response. I fixated on the text box but did not reply. I wondered if he had more to say. I hoped he would explain his answer, but I was not prepared for his next response.

"I would do anything to have my wife back."

Three little dots lit up, indicating he was continuing to type.

"She died from her AVM, and I cry my sons to sleep every night."

I waited for more dots to illuminate but none appeared. Tears bubbled up in the corners of my eyes.

I blinked a few times to clear my tears. More dots. He shared more.

"She had brown hair and olive skin tone. She didn't know, no one knew, she had a brain tangle, nor had they ever heard of an AVM, until it killed her. There was no warning. It ruptured, and she died. Just like that.

We wish we would have known. I would have done anything to save her."

Then he told me the date of her birthday.

I sat straight up in bed with a jolt that frightened our sleeping dog. This man's beloved wife and I share the same birthday, St. Patrick's Day, the luckiest day of the year. And our children were the same ages, 5 and 3. I wanted to wake up my husband and shake him. I wanted to yell, to tell him how I felt sad and simultaneously ashamed and ungrateful. It was not fair to this man that when doctors discovered my AVM, my husband comforted me. It was not fair to this man that once when I thought my brain exploded, it was merely a panic attack. It was not fair that I lay alive next to my husband, still unsure about a credible treatment option from a world-renowned neurovascular surgeon, while this man slept alone.

For a moment, I wished I had died instead of her. She didn't deserve to die, and I wasn't sure how or why doctors incidentally found my AVM before it ruptured. None of it made sense. Why her and not me?

I blankly stared at the screen, still unable to reply, drowning in my own tears, suffocating in my spoiled world filled with love, support, and second chances. This man and I were online in the middle of the night to discuss the same affliction, but our situations were vastly different. His wife, the mother of his kids, was dead.

I felt the worst kind of survivor's guilt that night. I wasn't a survivor yet, but I had the chance to attempt survival that she never had.

I finally replied. "I am so sorry. I wish I had words to give you peace. This is not fair, and I am so mad at myself that I feel scared to have brain surgery." I worried my words were not kind, loving, or compassionate enough to comfort this man in the dark.

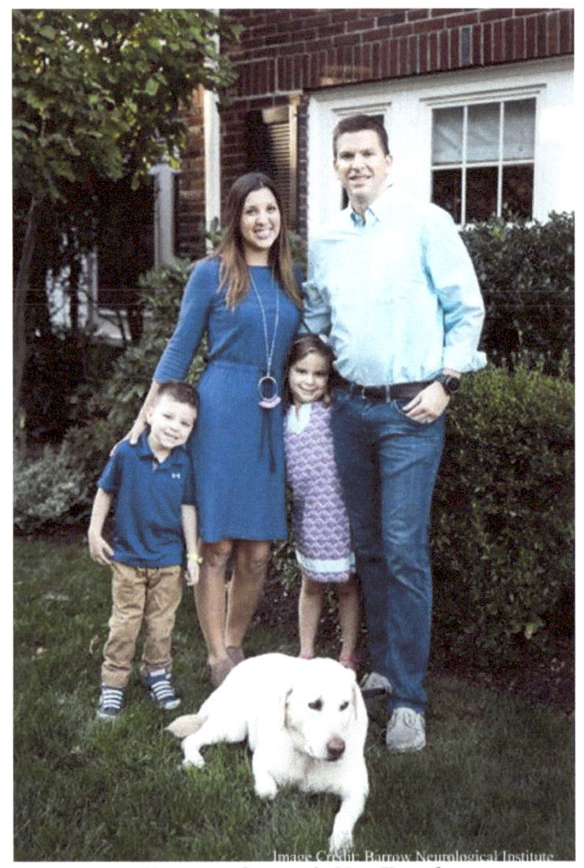

Vanessa Garza & Her Family

I waited a moment, then I saw the three dots again as his words materialized on my screen. "You should seek treatment if you trust your doctor. Your family wants you to be with them. And someday your kids will understand you did this for them. You are strong. I just hope I am strong enough for my boys, because I know she would be strong for them."

I closed my eyes for a few seconds, taking in his words. I felt the soft pillow behind my back and the warm blanket over my legs and cried a bit more. I finally wrote, "You are strong, and I know you are a great dad. Please know that I send your family all my love and best wishes. I will celebrate your wife every March, always. May she rest in peace."

I didn't know what else to say, and he did not respond again. I scrolled through our typed conversation in disbelief and re-read the words about March birthdays, young children, and brain bleeds. I looked over at my husband and adjusted the blankets to cover his left shoulder. Although I cried myself to sleep, I knew my tears did not compare to a widower's in mourning.

> **Although I cried myself to sleep, I knew my tears did not compare to a widower's in mourning.**

What if I had died from my AVM and she lived instead? I envisioned my babies crying, sleeping in my husband's armpit nook, still crusty and blue from my favorite deodorant. I wondered if they would sleep on my side of the bed or if they would leave a space for me. How long would my pillow smell like my shampoo? Would they be angry if they knew I had a chance to remove my AVM, but chose not to undergo surgery because I was afraid?

The man I met in the dark changed my life and set me on a course, an uncertain course, to remove my AVM. He showed me that discovering my AVM before it hemorrhaged was not a misfortune; it was an opportunity to live. My decision to elect multiple brain surgeries became clear. I knew surgery would be risky, but I had to move forward for my family, and for his family too.

I went back to see that doctor. Four brain surgeries later, I am now AVM-free without complications, thanks to a man in the dark, and his wife in the light.

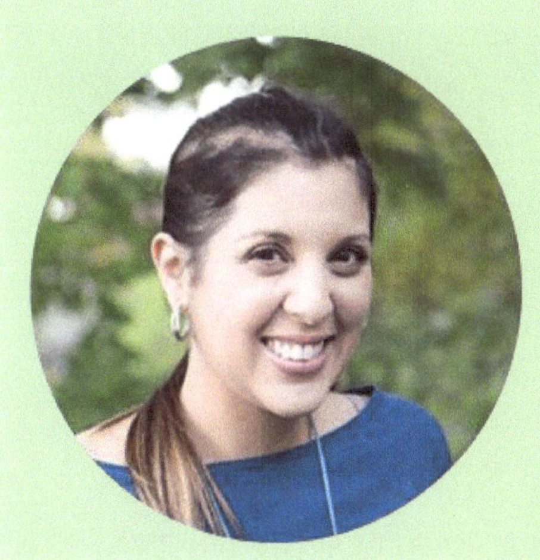

Meet Vanessa Garza

Vanessa is a Boston-based novice writer, mother, former corporate America consultant, and survivor of a brain arteriovenous malformation (AVM), a very rare neurological condition. In the summer of 2017, she elected to have four brain surgeries to remove the AVM. Thanks to successful therapies and her newly minted brain, secured with titanium plates and screws, she is motivated to heal, recover, and write. She hopes to inspire anyone at risk for stroke, to raise awareness for this very rare neurological disease, as well as to honor all TBI warriors with both good and devastating outcomes.

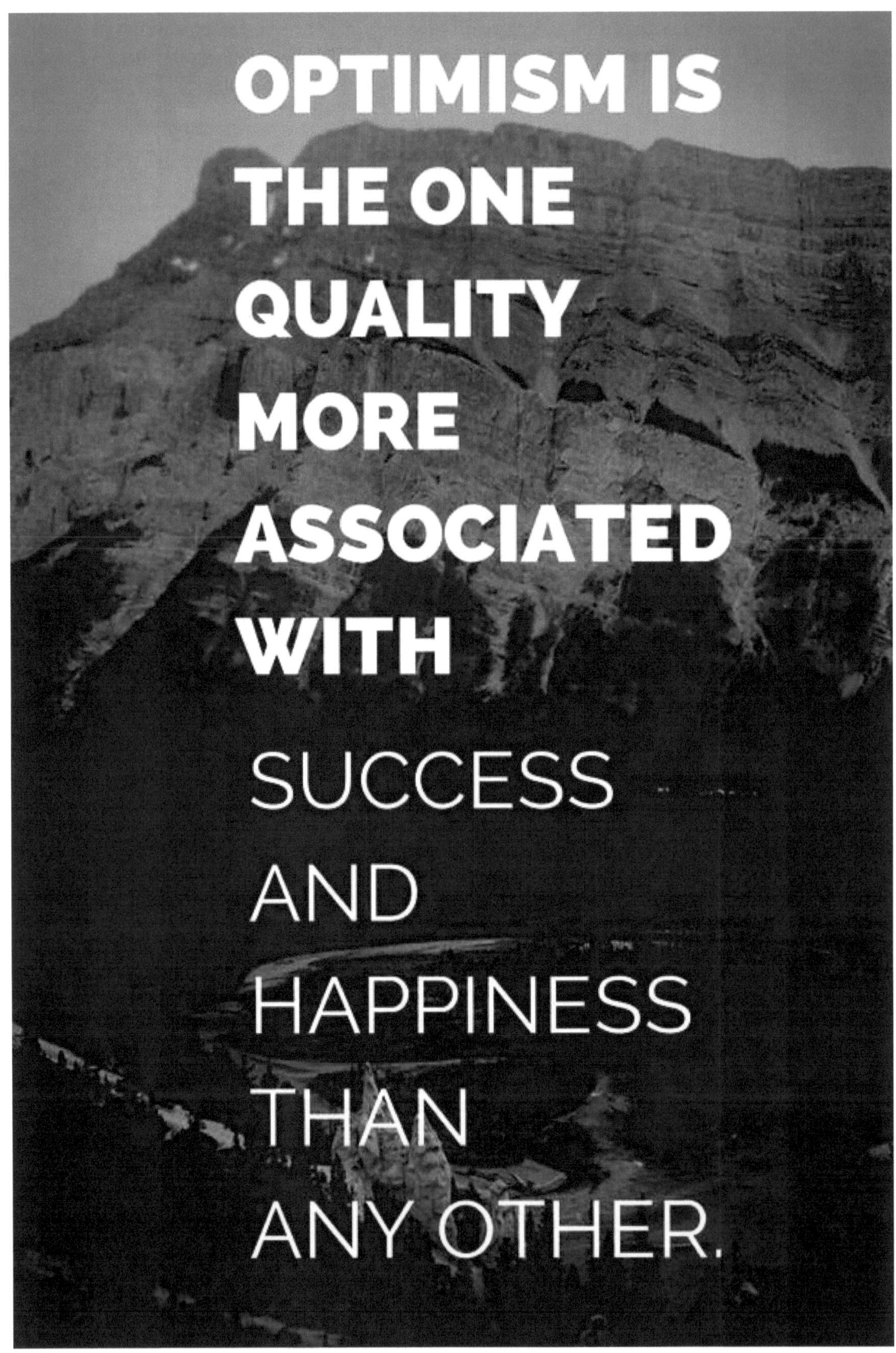

OPTIMISM IS THE ONE QUALITY MORE ASSOCIATED WITH
SUCCESS AND HAPPINESS THAN ANY OTHER.

It's Okay to Let Go

By Martin Johnson

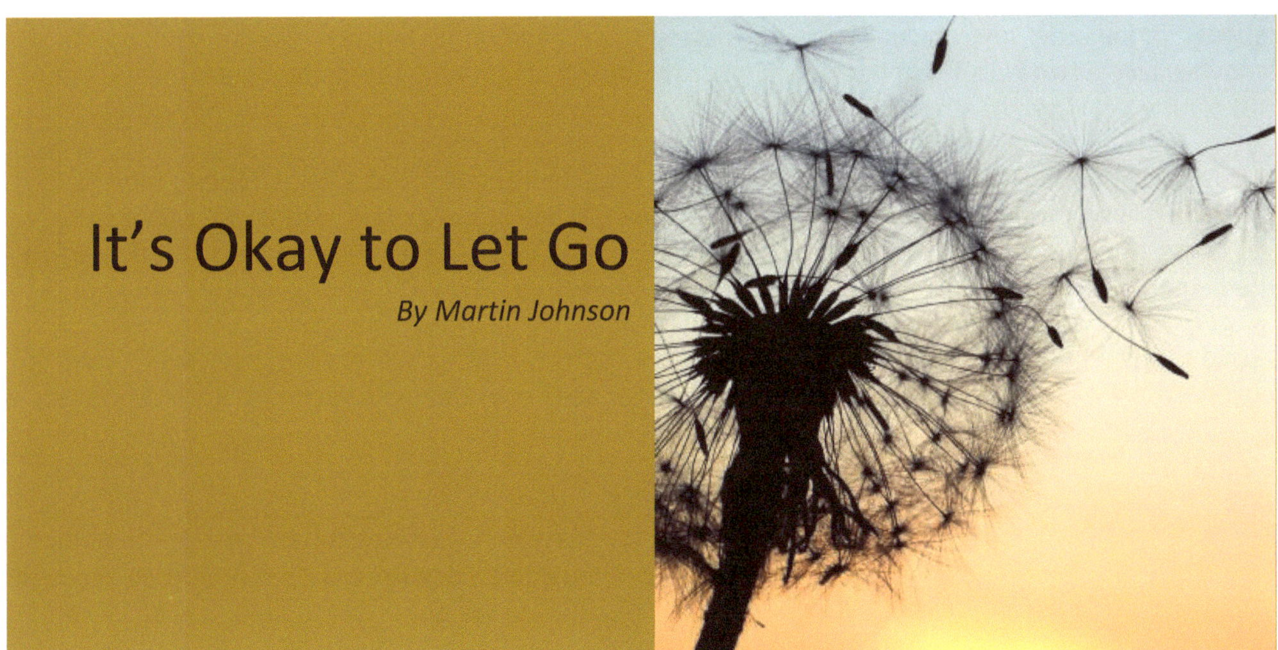

The nineteen-nineties started well for me. By the mid-nineties, I thought I was on top of the world. I had a good job and was an English major in college. I was the life of the party in my social circles.

Being ambidextrous made me an avid gamer everyone wanted to watch and helped me to be a decent guitar player. I lived life a little too fast because I thought nothing could stop me.

All of this came to a crashing halt the day before Easter in 1997. I was involved in a severe car accident that left me with an open head injury. During emergency brain surgery, I suffered fifteen mini-strokes and pretty much died.

After miraculously surviving, the doctors performed a partial frontal lobe lobotomy to remove the damaged part of my brain. Of course, all of this was unbeknownst to me until about a week later when I woke up to my new life.

> *"The left side of my face drooped, I had lost the fine-tuned motor skills in my left hand, I talked monotone like a real-life Forest Gump, and I could barely walk."*

At first, it seemed like a nightmare, everything I had worked so hard for was gone. The damage to the right side of my brain had partially paralyzed the left side of my body. The left side of my face drooped, I had lost the fine-tuned motor skills in my left hand, I talked monotone like a real-life Forest Gump, and I could barely walk.

But it wasn't the end of my story, just the beginning of a new way of living. I still have many more chapters to live and to write. Of course, it is a different story, but it is still my story.

About a month after my accident I was transferred to a rehabilitation hospital. I was wheeled in on a stretcher face down because my paralysis made me unable to get onto the stretcher and I could only roll off my bed onto the stretcher.

It was there I first learned about my lack of feeling and control of my left side. After two months of grueling rehabilitation, I was allowed to go home and do outpatient therapy. However, playing the guitar and gaming were no longer options. At that point, I decided to give up on what I used to do and tried embracing the new life I had.

I tried riding a bike only to fall off. Determined to be active, I started cutting the grass with a push lawnmower for hours every day to regain my strength and conditioning. Eventually, I was biking a 21-mile route in the heat of summer.

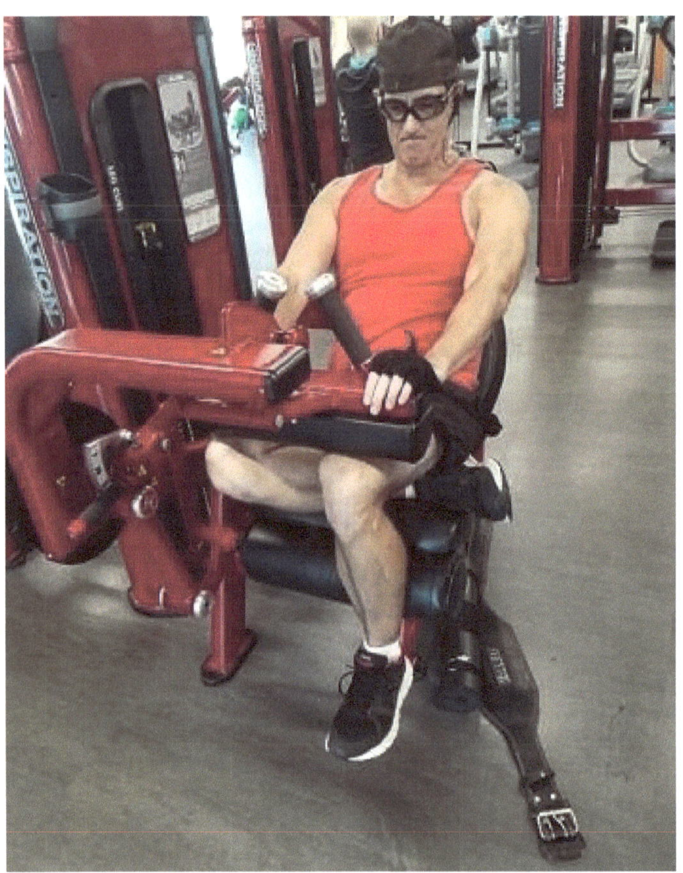
Martin Working Out

About a year later I continued my recovery process by joining a local gym to strengthen the left side of my body. I progressed enough that I was noticed by a modeling scout and soon I was modeling as a high-fashion and fitness model in Atlanta.

While most of my college friends were graduating from college, partying and playing games. I was learning to accept that my life was different. In hindsight, I've never looked back and for the most part, I don't miss the old me.

I've learned that when a door closes, stop knocking on it and look for another door that may open. After ten years of modeling and working as an extra in Atlanta, my agent died unexpectedly.

That door closed, and then I was allowed to take part in a professional writing program. During those four years, I learned the skills and traits needed to pursue a professional writing career.

Since then I've written an award-winning screenplay about a college student who suffers a TBI after 9/11. As well as writing numerous articles and nine books I'm currently seeking representation for, I continue to speak to other brain injury survivors and share what I've learned over the last twenty-two years. I currently write a monthly blog and two columns for a writing website.

Through my writing and speaking, I get to share my story of how living with a disability challenges me and changed me but didn't kill me. I still bike and work out and I'm in better shape physically than most people half my age. My workouts are not for superficial reasons, but to help keep atrophy and other side effects of brain injuries from setting in.

One of my quirks is I can't sit still long, I'm reminded of those early days being confined to a wheelchair, one I couldn't even move on my own because I couldn't feel my left arm. I was completely dependent on other people to push me around; it was humiliating, to say the least, and I am grateful for having the physical abilities I have regained. Now, I take advantage of every opportunity I get to be active.

The things I enjoy doing now are not what I used to do and honestly never thought I would enjoy. But, being disabled has become my new normal, I no longer grieve the things I've lost due to my disability, only because I've learned its okay to let go.

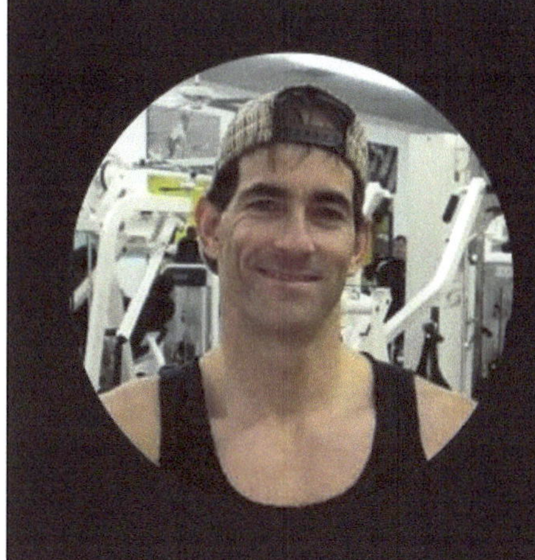

Meet Martin Johnson

Martin Johnson is an award-winning writer, columnist, speaker and brain injury advocate located in Georgia. He has lived with a severe brain injury for almost 23 years and understands the trials and setbacks of living with a brain injury. When not writing or helping others with disabilities, you can find him in the local gym or outside being active. He is determined to not let losing 30% of his brain after a car accident hold him back. Martin's brain was injured in a car accident in 1997 and underwent a frontal lobe lobotomy to remove the damaged side of his frontal lobe. Even with a lack of feeling on the left side of his body, he knows life must go on.

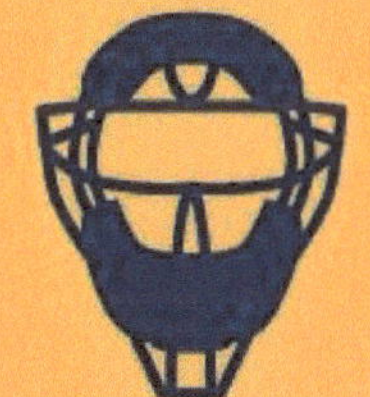
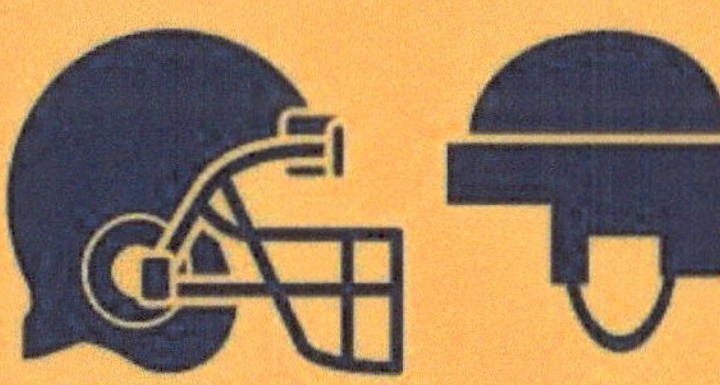

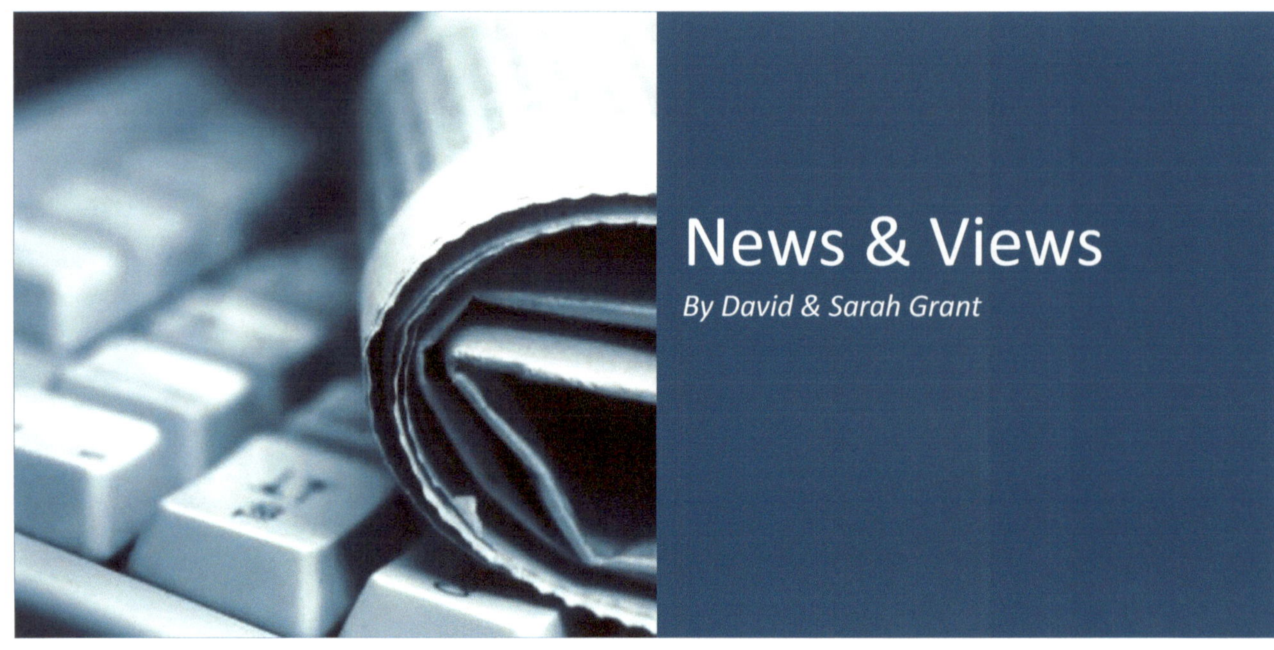

Looking back over the hundreds of articles we've published since 2013, it's amazing to see how much we've changed as a brain injury resource.

Those readers who have been with us since the beginning will recall the first itteration of our publication: *TBI Hope and Inspiration*. At the time, we naively thought that all brain injuries were traumatic brain injuries.

As the years passed, we continued to learn, and change both the name of our publication as well as the stories that we now feature. This month's issue is a perfect example. You've just read stories by traumatic brain injury survivors, an AVM survivor, as well as a "raw and real" submission by a caregiver.

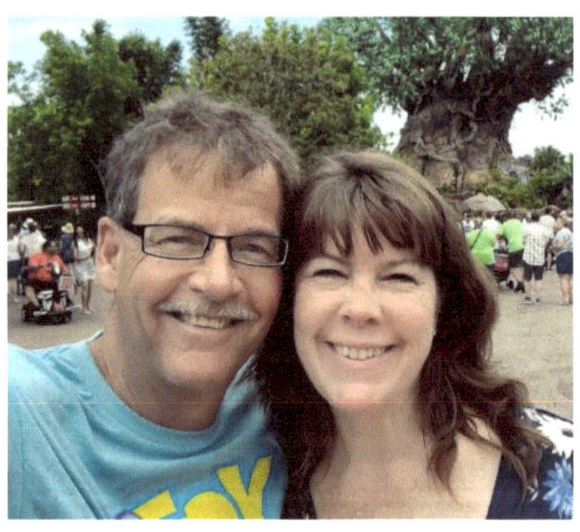

As we move forward, we have grown in terms of the diversity of voices now heard in HOPE Magazine. And it is with that diversity that we strive to offer even more people the opportunity to see that they are not alone – and that others not only share their fate, but more importantly, have found a way to live meaningful lives.

Peace,

~David & Sarah